WHEN EVERY BITE MATTERS

One Teen's Journey with Food Allergies

OLIVIER DELDICQUE

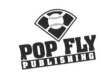

POP FLY
PUBLISHING

FAYETTEVILLE, NEW YORK

When Every Bite Matters
One Teen's Journey with Food Allergies

Copyright © 2018 by Olivier Deldicque

POP FLY PUBLISHING
508 Briar Brook Run
Fayetteville, NY 13066

For more information please visit: **PopFlyPublishing.com**

Published in the United States of America

Paperback ISBN: 978-0-578-41853-7
eBook ISBN: 978-1-5323-9437-9

Cover and author photograph: **Epoch Photography, Epochpic.co**

Book design and layout: **Shannon Bodie, BookWiseDesign.com**

HI THERE!

Before you read this book, remember, I'm a teenager, not a doctor! This book does not take the place of medical advice from your allergist or doctor. I've made every effort to ensure that the content provided in this book is accurate and helpful to readers. Much of it is based on my own experiences and opinions. Always talk to your doctor about how you manage your allergies.

No liability is assumed due to the information provided here, nor do I claim responsibility for adverse effects resulting from the use of recipes and/or information found within this book.

—O.D.

CONTENTS

FOREWORD

I was excited to read this brave story told by a remarkable young man. Fifteen-year-old Olivier Deldicque was first diagnosed with a life-threatening allergy to milk when he was four months old. He also has allergies to peanut, tree nuts, raw egg, and some fish. In this eye-opening book, he speaks about the challenges of life with food allergies, but also about sports, cooking and travel—passions that he engages in safely by knowing the risks, planning in advance and being aware. By sharing his story and his positive attitude, Olivier offers advice, inspiration and empathy to kids growing up with food allergies, their families, and friends and neighbors who don't yet understand this life-changing and increasingly common disease.

Olivier is one of many exceptional teens with food allergies who I've had the pleasure to meet as the CEO of Food Allergy Research & Education (FARE). Our organization is committed to helping these young people find their voice and advocate for themselves. Their stories, like this one, powerfully illustrate the courage it takes to remain aware of constant hazards, but still live fully. I am confident that by telling their experiences in their own words, Olivier and others will help engage public support for the research, education and awareness efforts we need to reverse the rise of food allergy.

—LISA GABLE
CEO, Food Allergy Research
& Education (FARE)

FARE does not endorse the contents of publications authored by private individuals.

INTRODUCTION

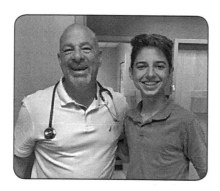

It is my great honor to introduce Olivier, and in reality his whole family, as they discuss their management and 'struggle' with food allergies. They have taken a potentially disabling and anxiety-provoking disorder and turned it into a positive, structured approach to his (their) disease. They have given a blueprint for others to follow. It is remarkable that at this young age, Olivier has achieved amazing maturity. His family is also to be congratulated on the balance that it has adapted. It also shows that withdrawal and restrictions to lifestyle aren't recommended in dealing with food allergies. I have followed the Deldicque brothers since they moved here from Connecticut in 2008. At first the boys were shy and somewhat reserved around me, but they have grown up to be remarkable young men who have become advocates for their disorder, which is so prevalent and has risen in almost epidemic proportions. I hope you enjoy their journey and use their experience as a platform for change and education for those families dealing with fears and their own struggles with food allergies, as I have!

—JUAN L. SOTOMAYOR, M.D.
Allergy, Asthma & Immunology
Board Certified in Pediatrics
& Allergy/Immunology

PROLOGUE

It was a warm summer day in August. My mom, my brothers, and I were shopping at Barnes and Noble. We all picked out books (I chose *The Maze Runner*) and went to get a drink at the store's cafe. I love the banana chocolate shakes—yum!

My brothers and I were kidding around waiting for our drinks. They called our order, and I received my shake along with my brother's chocolate milk. I gave him the milk, and we sat down with our mom to have our drinks.

We were talking when I began to have a strange feeling. I took another sip of my delicious drink, when suddenly my mouth began to tingle. Within a couple of seconds the all-too-familiar itching started on the roof of my mouth. My throat began to feel swollen.

I knew in a few minutes I wouldn't be able to breathe...

ALL ABOUT ME

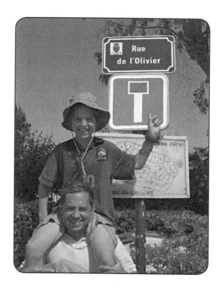

My name is Olivier Francis Deldicque. Not Oliver. Maybe you haven't heard the name before because it's French. My dad, Greg, is from France, but it was actually my mom who chose my name. I'm told my grandpa from Missouri wasn't too thrilled when he heard the choice.

My dad is laid-back and "go with the flow." He has a French accent, so sometimes it's funny when he talks. He is a businessman who travels a lot for work.

We live in Syracuse, one of the snowiest places in the U.S., so I ski a lot with my dad in the winter.

My mom, Alison, on the other hand, is from Missouri. She is adventurous, nice, and supportive of my schoolwork. My mom is an exceptional chef, which is probably why I love food so much.

I'm the oldest of three brothers. My youngest brother, Sebastian, is eleven years old. He loves spending his free time playing with Legos or with his wrestler action figures. His favorite wrestler is Kofi Kingston. Sebastian also plays basketball and is completely addicted to his iPad. He is generous, outgoing, and smart.

My other brother, Mathias, is fourteen years old. He is a very fast runner but is most passionate about basketball and loves the Cleveland Cavaliers. He also likes Legos and wrestlers. Currently, his obsession is with his collection of Kendama cup-and-ball games. Mathias is energetic, dramatic, and also kind.

As for me, I'm fifteen. I was born in Los Angeles (in the same hospital where Shaquille O'Neal's son was born a few days before!), but I don't remember a single thing from the nine months I lived there. After that, my dad got a job in Connecticut where we lived until I was six. When I was about to start kindergarten, we moved to Syracuse, New York, where we still live today.

I love my brownish-blackish hair that I spike up. I'm pretty tall for my age. In my free time, I love to listen to and mix music, and I've even DJ'ed for a couple of parties. My favorite artists are Drake, Jeremih, and Bruno Mars.

I also like to play the drums and sing and dance, so I've been doing theatre since I was four years old. I've performed in approximately eighteen shows with Syracuse Children's Theatre including playing Troy in *High School Musical*. That show was especially fun because I could play basketball on stage. Recently, I played Conrad Birdie in the show *Bye Bye Birdie* at my high school. That production was so fun!

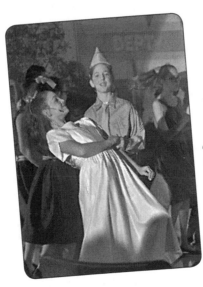

ONSTAGE AS
CONRAD BIRDIE

When I'm not in class, I enjoy working out, biking, skiing, playing sports like basketball, and competing on my school's soccer and track teams.

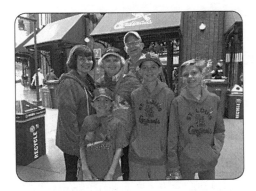

GO CARDINALS!
AUNTIE CAROLYN,
NANA, PAPA,
SEBASTIAN, ME,
AND MATHIAS IN
ST. LOUIS.

My mom is from "Cardinal Nation," so baseball is in my blood. Everyone in my family is a major St. Louis Cardinals fan, especially me. Even my French dad has grown to like baseball. I went to my first Major League Baseball (MLB) game in San Diego when I was about four months old. My mom takes my brothers and me to a lot of games. In fact, I've been to twenty-one MLB stadiums so far. Plus, we're lucky to live close to the Baseball Hall of Fame in Cooperstown, New York, so we've been there a few times. I played Little League for many years, but now I just play for fun. I love to play Wiffle ball in the summer with my neighbors.

When we were at a Texas Rangers game four years ago, Prince Fielder was up to bat and hit a foul ball that hit my brother Mathias. He went to the hospital and seemed fine until the morning when he started throwing up. He had a concussion. It was horrible because he couldn't do anything for a while, and Mathias doesn't like to sit still! When we got home, the Rangers sent him a bat with all the players' signatures on it and the lineup sheet from the dugout. At least he got some souvenirs.

My brothers and I normally play on the Xbox (I love *NBA 2K18*) or play sports outside. On the weekends, I like to play on my phone and play Clash Royale, Brawl Stars, Clash of Clans, and check out my social media accounts. My family plays a lot of board games, too, which can get pretty competitive.

I also love to cook because I love to eat! My favorite recipes to make are pasta, quesadillas, and empanadas. I'll talk more about this later in the book.

Another thing I love and that I'm lucky to do is travel. I've traveled to France, England, the Dominican Republic, Canada, Argentina, Guadeloupe, Uruguay, Belgium, Monaco, Italy, Spain, and the Netherlands.

My family is Catholic, and we go to church every week. I also go to a Catholic school: Christian Brothers Academy. We live in a pretty normal neighborhood in the suburbs.

As you can see, my life is normal except for one thing: I have deadly food allergies. I'm severely allergic to milk, peanuts, raw eggs, and some kinds of fish. No milk means no butter, yogurt, ice cream, or cheese. Every time I eat something, I'm risking my life. For example, if I accidentally drink a sip of cow's milk or eat a spoonful of dairy yogurt, my throat will close up and I won't be able to breathe.

I don't remember my first allergic reaction because

I was four months old, but my parents certainly do. I know it was tough for them because it's frightening to see your newborn child having an allergic reaction. My mom is going to tell you how it happened:

I was overjoyed to become a mom when Olivier was born! Right after his birth, though, I was sick and Olivier was taken care of in the hospital's nursery. He drank bottles of milk-based formula. After that, I took care of feeding him.

One night, when he was about four months old, Olivier's dad, Greg, gave him a bottle of milk-based formula and put him to bed. We had a baby monitor, the old-fashioned kind you plugged into the wall that had a little speaker.

After Greg came downstairs, we heard Olivier on the speaker making some strange noises. He wasn't crying, but something didn't sound right. Greg went up to his room to check on him. A little while later, I went up to the nursery, where Greg was standing, holding Olivier in the dark.

"I can't get him settled," Greg said.

"Bring him over here, into the light," I requested.

When Greg stepped into the light, I could see.

"Greg, Olivier's covered in hives!"

Greg and I were new parents, and we were scared. We called the pediatrician first, but she told us to take Olivier to the hospital. We all thought it was some kind of reaction, and it sounded like Olivier was having trouble breathing.

Fortunately, Cedars-Sinai Medical Center was right down the street from us in Los Angeles. We arrived in the emergency room and were immediately taken back to a big room, even though there were a lot of people waiting. I was scared. My little baby was all red and covered in hives.

A team of doctors and nurses put Olivier on a big metal table. It felt like we were in an operating room. There was equipment everywhere. Olivier looked so small lying there. Amazingly, he wasn't even crying.

The doctors gave Olivier an injection of epinephrine and checked him over carefully. Based on the information we provided, the doctors seemed fairly certain he'd had an allergic reaction to milk.

Even though he had had cow's milk when he was first born, he hadn't drunk any for several months, until that evening. Several hours later, we took Olivier home with instructions to see an allergist as soon as possible.

A few days later, we met Olivier's first allergist. He was very kind and answered all our questions. Greg and I didn't understand how Olivier could be allergic to milk. We didn't have any allergies. Plus, I was nursing Olivier, and I ate a fair amount of dairy. The doctor did a blood test—Olivier cried that time—that later confirmed our baby boy had a life-threatening allergy to milk.

Knowing what we know now, we realize how lucky

we had been. If we hadn't gone back up to check Olivier that night, he could have died. If we hadn't made it to the hospital in time, he could have died. Instead, he was alive and well. He wasn't eating solid foods yet, so Greg and I had a little time to prepare for the non-dairy diet Olivier's life would depend on. We didn't know yet that Olivier was allergic to other foods as well...

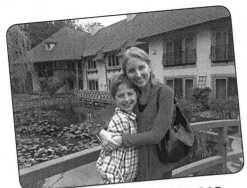

MY MOM LIKES TO REMEMBER
THE GOOD OLD DAYS WHEN SHE
WAS TALLER THAN ME!

And that's how it all began. About that same time, I started to have severe *eczema*. Eczema is an itchy skin rash that's hard to treat. Even though we lived in California, I had to wear long sleeves all the time because I scratched my skin until it bled. My parents and my dermatologist tried everything to figure out what was causing it. I do remember taking oatmeal baths for years. We believe the eczema had something to do with my allergies. It lasted several years until suddenly it disappeared. It still drives my mom crazy that she never figured out what was causing it.

As I said earlier, we moved to Connecticut when I was nine months old. My first memories are of living there. My allergist's name in Connecticut was Dr. Mendelson. He always had lollipops in his pocket and little animals clipped to his stethoscope. He monitored my food allergies, and it turned out I was also allergic to eggs, nuts, and some fish. Around this time, I started preschool with my best friend, Sam. Sam would never bring peanut butter because he knew about my allergies and wanted to be able to sit next to me. All these years later, he's still one of my best friends.

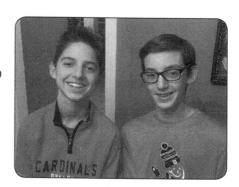

SAM (ON THE RIGHT) AND I HAVE BEEN FRIENDS SINCE WE WERE BABIES!

I remember that when kids in preschool had birthday treats, I couldn't eat them, so my teacher, Mrs. Claffey, would give me a Fruit Roll-Up or a candy Lego brick. It's funny the memories that stick with you.

When I was almost two, my brother Mathias was born. Since I had allergies, he was tested right away. In the beginning, Mathias was allergic to wheat, milk, eggs, and nuts. Fortunately, he outgrew the wheat, milk, and egg allergies, but he's still allergic to nuts.

A year after my other brother Sebastian (who doesn't have any allergies) was born, we moved to Syracuse just in time for me to start kindergarten. That's where we've been living ever since.

I think of myself as a normal teenager who happens to have food allergies. Through this book, I'll share my story, which I hope will help you manage your allergies and feel normal, too.

ALL ABOUT YOU:

Take a few minutes to think about your own "allergy story."

- When were you diagnosed with a food allergy?
- What are your first memories of having a food allergy?
- Does anyone else have a food allergy in your family?

OLIVIER'S FOOD ALLERGY BASICS

ALLERGY VS. INTOLERANCE

Some people confuse a food allergy with an intolerance. These are very different conditions. An *intolerance* is when you can't *digest* a food. It's most common with dairy but doesn't really happen with nuts. Some symptoms of an intolerance are bloating, passing gas, and having major stomach issues.

I'm sure a food intolerance is a pain, but it frustrates me when people call an intolerance an allergy. They are very different. One involves the digestive system, the other, the immune system. People won't die from an intolerance, but people could die from an actual food allergy.

WHAT IS A FOOD ALLERGY, EXACTLY?

Fifteen million Americans have food allergies.[1] Every one in thirteen children in the U.S. has a food allergy. In other words, there is probably someone suffering from allergies in every class you have at school. If you don't have an allergy, I'm sure you know someone who does. The latest study shows a 377% increase in anaphylactic food reactions from 2007 to 2016.[2]

A *food allergy* is when the body's immune system reacts to a certain food. The *immune system* is a network of cells, tissues, and organs that defends the body from viruses and other diseases. Our immune system's job is to fight off germs. If you have a strong immune system, you will not get sick as easily as a person with a weak immune system. I think about the immune system being an army inside my body. Every army has soldiers, and the body's soldiers are called antibodies. However, people with allergies in addition produce an allergic antibody called Immunoglobulin E (IgE). No one knows why.

Normally the immune system attacks germs, but in people with food allergies, the "soldiers" (antibodies) see a food like peanuts as an enemy attacking the body. Because of this, they fight back. This "reaction" to the food can be fierce and can cause symptoms like closing of the throat, hives, nausea, dizziness, difficulty breathing, rapid breathing, and fainting. If the immune system wages an all-out battle on the food, the person can have an anaphylactic reaction. This is what could be fatal.

Anaphylaxis is life-threatening. Let's talk more about how this can happen. Eating something your body is allergic to might lead to "anaphylactic shock." Suppose you are allergic to peanuts and you eat one. It will first go down your esophagus and then hit your respiratory system. The bronchial tissues will then get inflamed. You will start to have difficulty breathing. You might start to cough or wheeze.

If you do not treat this shock with a dose of epinephrine, you will die. The reaction also affects the central nervous system. You might feel a headache or dizziness, which might cause you to lose consciousness. Anaphylaxis also impacts the circulatory system. Your blood pressure can drop during anaphylactic shock. If you get low blood pressure, the organs in your body can't function well because your blood isn't circulating and delivering enough oxygen. Your heart could stop, and you might go into cardiac arrest. At the same time, it's probably wreaking havoc on your digestive system and you could start throwing up.

Anaphylaxis can happen in different ways, and it can happen VERY fast, in a matter of seconds. The ONLY way to stop it is with a dose of epinephrine.

MY LIFE-SAVING TOOL

Epinephrine is the same substance as adrenaline. *Adrenaline* is a hormone produced in our bodies. This hormone increases our heart rate so that we can do things we normally can't. You may have heard the phrase "fight or flight." These are the sorts of stressful situations where adrenaline kicks in. Adrenaline opens up airways so more oxygen gets to our muscles to help us out in emergency situations. Our body feels less pain when adrenaline is flowing through us, too. Adrenaline opens up the bronchioles in our lungs. You've probably felt an adrenaline rush before. For example, I sometimes get an adrenaline rush before I perform on stage. I can feel my heart pounding, and I feel like I could run around for hours.

When someone has an anaphylactic reaction, an injection of epinephrine can stop it because, much like an adrenaline rush, it opens up the airways in the lungs, decreases swelling, and increases blood pressure.

People like me with food allergies need to carry an auto-injector that contains epinephrine. The auto-injector contains a dose of epinephrine that a person can inject into their own leg. That thing saves lives! The most commonly known auto-injector is called the EpiPen®. Another newer brand is AUVI-Q®, which is shaped to fit in your pocket and has audio directions for its use.

Epinephrine is really a wonder drug from nature. It's the only drug that can reverse anaphylaxis. The mantra I always hear is "epi first, epi fast." It's critical not to wait in using your epinephrine because it may not be as effective.

Whenever you use the auto-injector, you must

also call 911. You need to call 911 so that paramedics can check your heart rate. It's also important because, for some people, one dose of epinephrine may not be enough. The allergic reaction could continue. It is estimated that a food allergy reaction sends someone to the emergency room every three minutes.[3]

Once, when I had to use the auto-injector, we called 911 and the ambulance came. The paramedics asked me what had happened and how I was doing. They made me breathe through a tube to check my breathing. I was doing okay. They put me in an ambulance to go to the hospital. On the way to the hospital, they gave me an IV with fluids that hurt very badly! It made my arm clench up, and my face turned red like a fireball. When we got to the hospital, I went to a room and the doctors helped me out.

Another reason to go to the hospital is in case of a delayed reaction. That's when someone seems to be fine because their symptoms have calmed down only to come back again.

There is another drug that can help with an allergic reaction: the antihistamine. Benadryl® is an antihistamine you've likely heard of. Histamines are chemicals that exist in everyone's bodies to fight off allergens. Histamines can make a person sneeze if they get pollen in their nose, for example. That's good, but the body can overreact and release too many histamines, which causes an allergic reaction. When I eat a food I'm allergic to, too many histamines get released. An antihistamine drug can reverse what the histamines are doing, so taking a Benadryl tablet can help relieve an itchy throat, swelling lips, and hives.

However, please note that an anaphylactic reaction can happen within seconds, and Benadryl cannot work that fast. It's for minor allergy symptoms and not to be used instead of epinephrine.

Allergic reactions are different for everyone. For instance, if I ingest nuts, I have to use the auto-injector immediately. However, if I have a tiny amount of milk, I only need Benadryl. If I have a lot of milk, I need to use the auto-injector. (I'll explain more about that later.) I carry both an epinephrine auto-injector and Benadryl with me wherever I go.

It's less common, but people can have allergic reactions to food without eating the food in question. I've heard about people having reactions to peanuts on airplanes (where there is poor air circulation), for example, if they are sitting near someone eating them. This doesn't happen to me. However, if I touch milk, or someone who just drank milk kisses my cheek, I will get hives.

People die every year from food allergies. These incidents can happen if someone eats something they don't know they're allergic to, if they mistakenly eat a dish that contains an allergen, or if someone doesn't have their auto-injector or doesn't use it fast enough. Sometimes a person might use their auto-injector, but if they have a major reaction, they still may not reach the hospital in time. The only real way to prevent a reaction is to not eat the food you're allergic to.

The biggest fear about having food allergies, at least for me and other allergy sufferers I know, is that we might die. I hear about these tragedies from my mom and from reading the news. I hear tragic stories of teens eating a food they thought was safe but the recipe had changed to contain their allergen. I hear about college kids who go to parties, eat food they're allergic to, don't have their auto-injector with them, and then by the time they get to the hospital, it's too late. Whenever I hear about this it worries me. I always wonder if I will die of an allergic reaction.

One problem, especially for teenagers, is that they think it's not cool to carry an auto-injector. I ALWAYS have mine with me no matter where I'm going. It has become a habit, the same as grabbing my phone before I leave the house. Maybe it's easier for me because I've had to do it my whole life.

Someone might not think I'm cool, but my auto-injector might save my life.

MY REACTIONS

An allergic reaction has many different symptoms. For me, a reaction usually starts with an itchy throat and hives on my wrist. Hives are little red bumps, kind of like mosquito bites, that form on your skin and itch. My throat will start to thicken up, the hives will spread, and then my stomach will start to hurt.

I've never had a reaction to nuts, thank goodness, but I've had numerous reactions to milk, eggs, fish, and cantaloupe, which I was allergic to for a short time. I've had to use my auto-injector three times in total.

The first time was when my mom packed dairy yogurt in my lunch when I was in third grade. It wasn't her fault, but she still feels terrible about it. It was a new yogurt our grocery store had started selling. The company makes both soy and dairy yogurt, and the cartons look exactly the same. They were next to each other on the shelf, and my mom bought the wrong one. I sat down at lunch with my friends and ate a few scoops of the yogurt.

All of a sudden, it happened. My mouth was ferocious with itchiness. I ran to the nurse, and she stabbed me with the auto-injector. It all happened so fast I didn't have much time to get scared. Luckily, I recovered quickly, but we never bought that brand of yogurt again!

Another time, my dad mistakenly gave me dairy milk at home. When I was young, my dad would always give me soy milk in the morning. He would also give my brothers dairy milk. One morning, he mixed up the cups, and I drank the dairy milk. That was

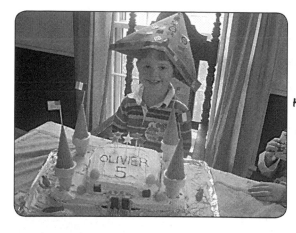

ALWAYS HOMEMADE BIRTHDAY CAKES FOR ME!!

horrible. When I was first diagnosed with food allergies, we didn't have dairy milk even in our house, but now we do. To be safe, we keep all the dairy products in a special part of the refrigerator.

The third time was almost three years ago when I was trying oral immunotherapy (OIT) at my allergist's office. (I will explain more about OIT later.) Remember how I said some reactions can be delayed? My mom and I were on our way home before I started to have a reaction to the milk. By the time we got home, it was severe enough that my mom needed to give me the auto-injector and call 911.

Besides these three instances, I've had plenty of smaller reactions over the years. When I get an allergic reaction, I concentrate on staying calm. I don't panic because then it could get worse. When I get a reaction, I don't get mad. (Most of the time.)

Many people fear using their auto-injector so they wait too long or don't use it at all. This misconception is dangerous and must be overcome and usually is after the first time you use it.

One thing I realized after using the auto-injector the first time is that it didn't hurt as badly as I expected. Think of the auto-injector as your best friend and don't fear it. I was always so worried about having to use it, but it was surprising how quickly it stopped my reaction.

YOUR FOOD ALLERGY BASICS:

- Do you have a friend or family member with a food allergy or intolerance? If so, what is he/she allergic to?

- Do you know what to do if they ingest the food they're allergic to?

- Do you know how to use an epinephrine auto-injector?

- If you have a food allergy, what happens if you ingest the food you're allergic to?

- Describe what it feels like when you have a reaction.

- Have you ever needed an epinephrine auto-injector? If so, describe this experience.

WHERE DO
FOOD ALLERGIES
COME FROM?

People ask me this all the time, and the answer is complicated. There is no clear explanation on how allergies develop. Most people find out they're allergic to something the hard way—by having a reaction. Others, like my brother, are tested for the most common allergens before ingesting them. Some people don't develop allergies until they are adults. A person could develop an allergy to a food they've eaten for years. For instance, my maternal grandfather developed an allergy to fish when he was an adult.

Food allergies are estimated to affect 4–6% of children according to the Centers for Disease Control and Prevention.[4]

I hear many adults say, "There weren't as many allergies back when we were kids." This is true. Allergies are on the rise. The Centers for Disease Control & Prevention report that the prevalence of food allergies in children increased 18% between 1997 and 2007.[5]

There are many theories on how you can develop a food allergy. Many people think that a food allergy is determined by genetics. In my family, there is no recollection of anyone having a food allergy before me except for my grandpa. Scientists don't know if genetics play a role or not. I think there may be something to do with it because my brother is allergic to nuts, too.

Another theory is that changes in the food supply are contributing to more allergies. Farmers are now using more chemicals and pesticides in their crops than they did before. Food companies also add chemicals and preservatives to a lot of the food we eat. People even use stronger chemicals and pesticides on their lawns. In Europe, fewer people have allergies, and many of the chemicals American farmers and food companies add to foods are illegal there. Based on this information, I believe there's definitely a correlation between chemical additives and allergies. Our bodies are not meant to be exposed to all of these artificial foods and chemicals. Not only that, but Americans also have a diet with more processed food and less fiber than in the past.

A third theory is that people are too clean. Nowadays, many people use antibacterial soaps, gels, and wipes regularly. Contrary to this behavior, many doctors and scientists think our bodies need to be exposed to some bacteria in order for our immune systems to work the right way.

This goes along with another idea about the overuse of antibiotics. Many farm animals are given antibiotics which then are in the food supply. Awareness is better now with this and doctors over prescribing antibiotics to patients. Again, this has an effect on the immune system.

No one knows if these theories are the true cause of food allergies or how they contribute to the development of food allergies. Many scientists are studying these ideas, testing theories and trying to develop treatments for food allergies. Hopefully we'll have clearer answers soon.

WHAT DO YOU THINK?

- Now that you know what I think, what are your ideas on where food allergies come from?
- If someone in your family has an allergy, do you think it plays a role in your own food allergy?

"WHAT CAN YOU EAT, OLIVIER?"

People ask me this question all the time, so let's get back to what I can and can't eat.

When I tell someone I have a dairy allergy, they think it must be hard for me to live an average, every-day life. It's true that I can't eat any food that contains milk, butter, cheese, etc. Most of these foods are off-limits to me:

- Cow's milk! (Of course.)
- Cupcakes, cakes, muffins, pies
- Cookies and brownies
- Ice cream
- Puddings (Most desserts, really!)
- Milkshakes
- Pizza
- Yogurt
- Whipped cream
- Pancakes, French toast
- Eggs prepared with milk or cheese

- Mashed potatoes
- Macaroni and cheese or any pasta with cheese
- Any salad with cheese or with a dressing containing dairy
- Any sandwich with cheese or mayonnaise
- Any cereals, crackers, or chips that contain milk
- Anything cooked with butter, like vegetables, meats, or fish

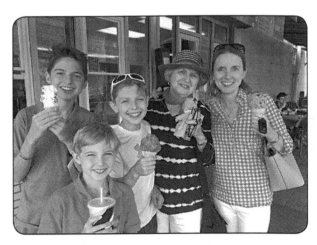

HERE I AM WITH MY BROTHERS, NANA, AND MOM. OUR LOCAL ICE CREAM SHOP, GANNON'S, IS VERY ATTENTIVE TO ALLERGIES. IN THIS PHOTO, I'M HAVING A NON-DAIRY ICE CREAM WITH SPRINKLES!

With my nut allergy, I can't have peanuts, almonds, cashews, tree nuts, or any other nut. That adds to the list of no-nos:

- Nuts and nut butter
- Nut milks
- Many cereals
- Granola bars
- Candy bars
- Many stir-fried Asian dishes
- Cookies and many of the desserts I've already mentioned

I'm also allergic to some fish, such as catfish and tilapia.

It looks like a big list of "NO's," doesn't it? Although it may seem like I can't eat much, I actually can. It really isn't bad because I've learned to live with my allergies and look for new, safe products at the grocery store.

The good news is, I can eat these foods without a problem:

- Fruits
- Vegetables
- Meats
- Some fish
- Other seafood

- Cooked eggs
- Grains

Also, many of the foods on my lists of no-nos can be prepared with substituted ingredients. My mom cooks and bakes food that is safe for me. We substitute soy milk in our pancakes and mashed potatoes at home, for example. Many restaurants can even prepare food that is safe for me to eat. For example, when I'm out with friends or family, I order pizza with no cheese.

Even better news is that, over time, companies have started making more dairy- and nut-free products to meet customer demand. For instance, I drink soy and coconut milk. I can eat ice cream and yogurt made from these milks, and I eat non-dairy cheese, which I can put on pizza, sandwiches, quesadillas, and pasta at home. There are a few brands of cookies and granola bars that are safe, too.

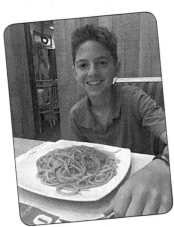

A LIFELONG DREAM: EATING PASTA IN ROME, ITALY!

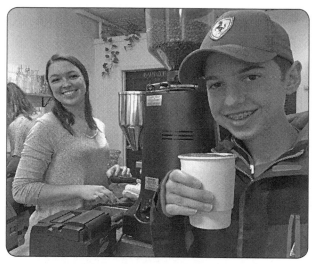

MY LOCAL COFFEE SHOP, SOLEIL, MAKES
ME A DAIRY FREE HOT CHOCOLATE
JUST HOW I LIKE IT!

WHAT CAN YOU EAT???

- Make a list of all the foods you're not able to eat and another list of foods that you CAN eat.

- Which list is longer? Circle the foods you really wish you could eat. Is there a way the recipe can be modified so that it doesn't contain things you're allergic to?

- How difficult is it for you to eat safe foods that you love? Do you enjoy food even though you have food allergies?

WILL I "OUTGROW" MY ALLERGIES?

Even though I am severely allergic to foods, I have made some progress over the years. As I said, at one point, I was allergic to cantaloupe, but I'm not anymore. I was also allergic to eggs. Now I can eat cooked eggs, but not raw ones (in mayonnaise or meringue, for example).

There is no cure for food allergies, but there is something called *desensitization* that can help. This is when you try to get your body used to the allergen, so it stops recognizing it as the enemy and stops reacting to it.

A few years ago, I tried an *OIT protocol*. OIT stands for oral immunotherapy. It's when you try to eat an allergen and expose your immune system to it little by little. For ten months, I went to my allergist once a week to try to reduce my dairy allergy.

I began with one tiny drop of milk diluted in water. I was extremely scared at first because I was literally drinking my poison. Every week I went back for a little more milk. If I felt a reaction, depending on how strong it was, I might have to drop down a couple stages, to a more diluted form of milk, or repeat the level again the next week.

I had my cocktail and then had to wait in the office so the doctor could monitor me. My mom knew how intense this was for me and took me every week to get a cinnamon sugar bagel when we finished. When I had my milk, it was stressful for me. Every time I drank the milk, I was putting the enemy inside my body. Drinking it gave me a weird sensation. Plus, it tasted horrible because I'm used to drinking soy milk.

After ten months, I was able to drink about a teaspoon of milk not diluted with water. One morning I had the milk and was fine and went to get my usual bagel. On the ride home, though, I began to have a serious delayed reaction.

It was so bad that I needed the EpiPen. We called 911, and the paramedics came. I went to the hospital and had to get an IV. I stayed there for a while to be monitored and then was fine. My body was finished with OIT.

My allergist and I talked about continuing the OIT for my dairy allergy, but going back to a much smaller amount of milk. I was very upset because I wanted to move forward and didn't want to take what I saw as steps backward. I had worked hard to get where I was.

My allergist also suggested a baked milk protocol. On this protocol, I would have a baked treat with a small amount of milk inside. This protocol worked! Now I can eat baked sweet treats if they contain smaller amounts of milk.

This made a huge difference in my life. For example, I don't have to worry about whether a hot dog bun has milk baked into it anymore. The most fun change my OIT protocol caused is that I can order a glazed doughnut at some places now!

I'm always hopeful about new therapies that are being tested, like the peanut patch—a "wearable patch that delivers small amounts of peanut protein through the skin"[6]—and other desensitization protocols. Researchers around the world work every day on solutions to treat allergies, which makes me hopeful about the future.

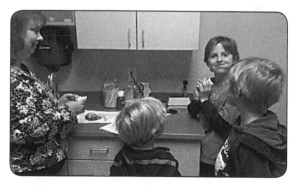

THAT'S ME A FEW YEARS AGO, EATING PART OF A MUFFIN IN MY ALLERGIST'S OFFICE.

When I'm at the allergist's office, I periodically have to get skin tests. During the skin tests, the doctors prick me with small drops of the foods I'm allergic to. If a hive appears, it means I'm still allergic to that food. If it looks like I have no reaction, the doctor might order a blood test or even a challenge test to see if my allergies have changed. For example, when my brother outgrew his dairy allergy, he went in and drank small amounts of milk over a few hours to be sure he had no reaction.

This is my scratch test from a few months ago. The big white bumps you see here are my reactions to cashews and pistachios.

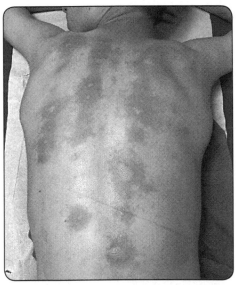

NOT MUCH PROGRESS THIS TIME. THOSE BIG CIRCLES ARE PISTACHIO AND CASHEW AFTER JUST A FEW MINUTES, AND YES, IT'S VERY UNCOMFORTABLE!!

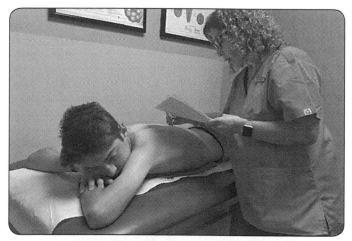

PRICKING THE SKIN WITH A TINY BIT OF
ALLERGENS IS A COMMON TEST

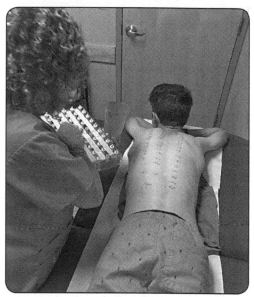

HOPING FOR IMPROVEMENTS ON THE SCRATCH
TEST IN MY ALLERGIST'S OFFICE.

ALL ABOUT YOU:

- How have your allergies changed over time?
- Have you talked with your doctor about participating in any desensitization protocols, like OIT?

MY LIFE WITH ALLERGIES

Life with allergies is different, but that doesn't mean it has to be difficult. That said, activities that are no-brainers for everyone else become dilemmas for kids with allergies: classroom parties, field trips, going out with friends, eating dinner at someone else's house. For some kids, even deciding what school to go to can be a challenge.

Here are several areas of my life and the way that I anticipate my needs related to food allergies in each situation. When it comes to your own life with allergies, work together with your parents and your support team to evaluate these situations on a case-by-case basis. Do what you feel comfortable with and not just what your parents are comfortable with. You arc the one with the allergies.

SCHOOL

Now that I'm in high school, I'm used to lockers and bell schedules. But when I moved from elementary to middle school, it was different for me in a lot of ways.

One of the changes you can probably relate to is now I have a block schedule and many teachers, instead of one homeroom teacher and a handful of resource teachers. In my elementary school, we stayed in one classroom for most of the day. My teacher always had my auto-injector with her, and the nurse's office had another one.

Now, at my new school, we switch classes, so I carry my auto-injector everywhere I go. (The nurse's office still has one, too.) This was a new responsibility for me, but I feel safer having it with me at all times. I never know when we may have an unexpected snack in one of my classes, or when my friends might eat candy or food I'm allergic to between classes.

At my old school, everyone knew about my allergies. My class was very small. There were only thirty people in my grade. My class was protective of my allergies because we had been going to school together for five years.

The biggest change for me, though, has been lunch period.

In elementary school, I always brought my lunch, but when I started middle school, I wanted to try eating in the cafeteria with all of my friends. Before the school year started, I went to campus and met with the chefs who make all the food in the cafeteria.

I felt a little nervous, but the cafeteria director

Kaylie was really nice. She knows the ingredients in everything the school serves and told me there were other kids with allergies, too.

Together we came up with a list of foods that are safe for me. Most days I eat chicken, French fries, fruit, or a salad. It felt very strange for the first month because I was used to bringing my own lunch, but in my new school, almost everyone eats the cafeteria food. Being able to eat cafeteria food makes me feel normal.

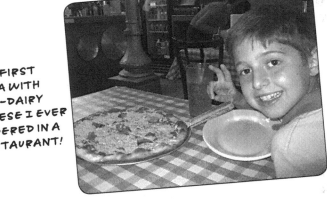

THE FIRST PIZZA WITH NON-DAIRY CHEESE I EVER ORDERED IN A RESTAURANT!

RESTAURANTS

As you might imagine, going out to eat is a challenge for people with food allergies. Every time I go to a restaurant, I have to ask if there is any dairy or nuts in the food I'm going to eat.

This has gotten a lot easier than it used to be because there's a lot more awareness of food allergies now. When I was younger, my parents ordered for me, and sometimes they'd get strange looks from the waiters and cooks.

Now that I'm older, I order for myself in restaurants. Whenever I order, I'm not afraid to say I have an allergy. At Chipotle, which uses an assembly line to prepare its food, I politely ask the person working to change their gloves before they start preparing my order. I can never be too careful if the person before me asked for cheese on their burrito!

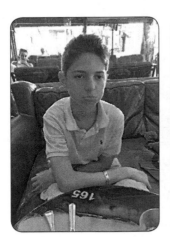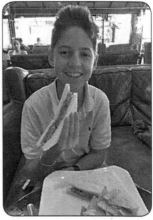

A LOT OF TIMES RESTAURANTS GET MY ORDER WRONG AND I HAVE TO SEND THE FOOD BACK. I'M USED TO BEING THE LAST PERSON TO GET THEIR FOOD!

And I can't just say, "Is there any dairy in that?" because the person might not understand that butter is dairy, for example. I usually make sure to ask if a meal has milk, cheese, or butter in it, depending on the food. Still, this process involves trust.

I also have to make sure I ask about cross-contamination. This means I have to make sure a food I order doesn't come into contact with a food I'm allergic to. In my case, if I'm ordering something grilled, I need to know whether the restaurant uses butter to grease the grill for other food. Of course, I always need to ask if food is fried in peanut oil, too.

Many restaurants now have allergen information available online or in store. Sometimes there are even special foods marked on the menu. For example, a lot of places have gluten-free sections or icons on their menu. I wish they had dairy-free, too!

Some states have laws about managing food allergies in restaurants. The latest information on these regulations can be found online in several places including Food Allergy Research & Education (FARE)'s website.

Of course, even being careful, mistakes may happen. Maybe the waiter or waitress doesn't hear the order clearly or they are handed the wrong food from the kitchen.

Because of this, my family is selective about where we eat. We avoid most Chinese and Thai restaurants because there are many nuts floating around, and sometimes a language barrier creates a potential allergy risk for me, too.

One summer in Florida, we were at a café, being served by a super-nice waitress. I ordered a turkey avocado wrap, and we discussed my allergies. We were sure to order the wrap without the mayonnaise.

My lunch came, and I started eating the delicious wrap. I was almost halfway finished when I began to feel funny. I looked inside the wrap and saw a huge clump of cheese! I immediately took some antihistamine. While we had been so careful about the mayonnaise, the menu didn't say the wrap had provolone cheese in it and the waitress didn't think of it. Luckily, I didn't eat enough to need my auto-injector, but it was close. The waitress felt terrible.

On that same trip, we had gone fishing and brought our fish to a restaurant to be cooked. Our whole family could tell right away that the waiter was not on top of things. We were very specific about having the fish cooked and asked about nuts and peanut oil in the kitchen.

After a little while, the waiter came out and told us he'd made a mistake. They'd put half of our fish in an oil that is also used to cook food with nuts. Well, since we'd caught our fish, it was not replaceable. We knew the rest of the fish would be plenty for us to eat, and we were grateful we learned this before my brother or I had eaten the contaminated fish. Still, the manager came out, apologized over and over again, and brought us free dishes of vegetables. They were really kind. I'm glad most places now "get it" with food allergies.

Something else I need to be mindful of when it comes to cross-contamination is ice cream shops. Many ice cream shops use the same scoopers to scoop out all of the ice cream. They typically rinse the scoop in between flavors, but this is not a safe enough cleaning process for me, or for anyone with a dairy or nut allergy. I only go to places that use separate scoopers for each ice cream and sorbet flavor, and again, I always assess the potential for cross-contamination.

While in some cases allergies can be so severe that it isn't safe to eat out anywhere, most people with food allergies can find somewhere they can enjoy a meal out and feel relatively safe.

If you are uncomfortable going out to a restaurant, another idea is to learn to cook. I love to cook! It helps me feel safe because I know exactly what I'm eating and that I won't have a reaction. There are many cookbooks available with allergen-free recipes. In fact, at the back of this book, I've included the names of my favorite cookbooks and some of my delicious, original recipes for you to try!

TRAVELING

Traveling is another big challenge when you have food allergies. Managing my brother's and my food allergies plays a big part in where we stay and what we eat when we vacation.

First of all, in many smaller airports there's no safe, healthy food to buy because the salads and sandwiches are all pre-made and have cheese or mayonnaise on them. It's so annoying because if I'm in a rush, I can't just grab something to eat besides gum, candy, chips, or Oreos.

Then, when I'm on an airplane it's super tough because if I have a reaction, there's no hospital nearby. Peanuts used to be a popular snack given out on airplanes. Now, it's not as common, and airlines have choices of snacks, like pretzels and cookies.

Even if the airline doesn't serve nuts, people can still bring them on the plane. It's really dangerous because if someone next to me is eating nuts and I accidentally touch one, I will have a skin reaction. Many planes now carry auto-injectors, but not all of them. Luckily, I've never have had to use the auto-injector on a plane.

When I travel, my mom nicely asks the crew if nuts will be served on our flight. (Although you can put this information into your reservation online, check with the gate agent because they rarely have the information.) Most of the time, when they find out about my brother's and my nut allergy, the airline won't serve nuts or they might ask the people around us to move to another seat if they're eating nuts.

We've never had anyone be rude to us before, but I've definitely heard stories where that hasn't been the case. My mom always says the key is to be polite because most people are understanding. My favorite airline right now is JetBlue. Not only do they not serve nuts, but they also have Chex Mix and nut-free cookies!!

When we board an airplane, my brother Mathias and I always wipe the tray table off and pack our own snacks and food. This is key because we never know if we might get stuck on a plane or delayed in an airport, much less if there will be food in those situations that we can eat.

Sometimes, like when we visit my father's family in France, we take overnight flights, which serve dinner. One trick my mom does on these flights is that she orders a kosher meal, a vegetarian meal, and the regular meals for us. Between those three meals, there is usually something safe for Mathias and me to eat. The kosher and vegetarian meals have food with labels a lot of times, but we never count on being able to eat airline food.

Once we get to our destination, there are other challenges. We normally go to France every summer to see my dad's family. France is a whole other allergy story that I'm going to have to write A LOT about.

There are not as many nuts in France, but cheese is very popular. Everywhere you go, there are cheese shops. Also, in France, they use butter on everything. And I mean everything! They put it on steak and vegetables, inside pastries and bread. France is mainly known for their bread. Sometimes, when we go to the bakery in France, there is butter in the bread and the croissants. Then I feel bad because my family doesn't want to enjoy these foods in front of me.

A few years ago, though, we found out that most of the olive bread in France is safe for me. My grandma buys me so much of it now! The stores there also have a "bio" section, which is like the organic or natural food areas of the grocery stores in the U.S. I've found really good soy puddings and some cookies with dark chocolate that are nut- and dairy-free, so I can survive and fulfill my chocolate cravings!

When we visit France, it's hard to ask if something has dairy because I don't speak fluent French. Luckily my dad is French, so he can speak to waiters, bakers, and cooks, and ask if I can eat their food. People don't tend to have as many allergies in France, so when we tell a French person about my allergies, they might not realize it's life-threatening. I worry they might think I'm a picky little American boy and not take the allergy seriously.

Managing allergies when you don't speak the language of the country you're visiting can be very

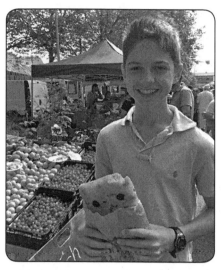

FINALLY FOUND SOME OLIVE BREAD
AT THE MARKET IN FRANCE!

dangerous. One thing that has proved helpful in the past is allergy cards. These are cards that describe your allergy in another language. They can be purchased or downloaded for free online. (You can find the link in this book, on the "Cool Resources" page.)

Every year my family goes to Club Med in Punta Cana in the Dominican Republic. The restaurants at Club Med are set up with food stations, and the chef who prepares the food stands there and serves it. This works well because they know all the ingredients. We meet with the head chef after arriving to review my and brother's allergies. Still, we walk through and have my parents help me choose food.

I recommend talking to a chef if you go to a restaurant or a resort like that. More and more, they are familiar with allergies and often have special desserts or substitute food available for people with food allergies.

Because I've found foods I can eat in France, I was surprised to find this wasn't the case when we went to Argentina for the first time. We could only find one brand of soy milk, and it took us forever to find it at a tiny market. There was no soy cheese or yogurt. (It's ironic because Argentina is a major producer of soy, and yet we could find NOTHING.)

Plus, in Argentina, some of the brands have different ingredients. Even though in the U.S. I can eat Lay's potato chips, in Argentina, they "may contain peanuts." Most of the chips and crackers were like that. I

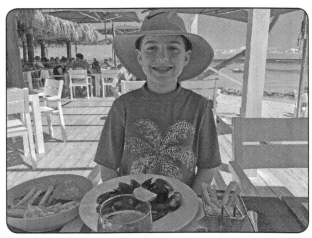

ALWAYS ORDERING CAREFULLY ON VACATION

had to be very careful the six weeks we were there. Most places serve meat, which is what Argentina is known for. (One point in Argentina's favor: they serve it grilled plain, without butter, which worked well for me.)

This summer we returned to Argentina, and I noticed even more changes in the labeling because the government has been working to improve labeling requirements. Before we arrived, my mom and I looked online and found some health food stores, and we emailed them to see if they carried soy milk. They were right around the corner from where I was taking Spanish classes!

If you are planning to travel, especially if you're going to a foreign country, I encourage you to do your research. Planning ahead can mean the difference between an enjoyable vacation and an ER visit in an unfamiliar place.

SOCIAL SITUATIONS

Of course, most parties have food, which is always an issue for someone with food allergies like me. My mom usually calls ahead to see what food will be served. Sometimes I bring my own cupcake or dessert since I never can eat birthday cake.

I have to really watch out when I go to a party. Even if I ask about a food, the person might not give me a correct answer because they aren't as used to reading labels. I'm not afraid to ask if I can see the package. People are always nice about it.

I also can't trust someone if they say they baked a cake or cookies without nuts or dairy. Even though they might try, unless they or their loved ones have food allergies, they will not be used to baking that way.

I heard a story once in which someone baked cookies without nuts and brought them to a party. However, the person had used the same utensil to remove peanut butter cookies from a pan earlier.

All of this to say, most people are relieved when I just bring my own dessert!

Last year, on the first day at my new school, there was a class party. Whenever I'm at a party and I see my friends eating brownies, cookies, and cakes, it feels strange to me. It feels strange because I see my friends eating what I can die from. It's like you're drinking water while all of your friends are drinking poison.

I'm grateful to have good friends, though. They always ask if it's okay if they eat something so they make sure I won't have a reaction. In my case, it's fine if someone is eating a food I'm allergic to as long as I don't touch it or, obviously, put it in my mouth. When I'm at a party, I don't get mad if my friends are eating stuff that I can't have. I've learned to deal with it and to be thankful for what I can have. At least I'm not allergic to soy or wheat like some people are.

Sometimes people worry whether or not they should invite a person with serious food allergies to a birthday party. Of course they should! We allergic kids like to have fun, too!

I go to sleepovers sometimes, but that can get dangerous. If someone does the whole "whipped cream in the hand" trick with me, I'll get a reaction. Because of this, I only go to sleepovers if my parents know the family well and the parents know how to use an auto-injector. Also, of course, I bring my own snacks.

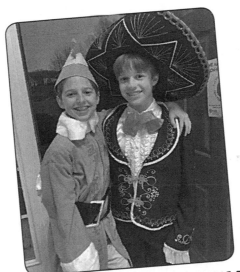

HALLOWEEN IS AN EVEN SCARIER TIME FOR KIDS WITH FOOD ALLERGIES. MY BEST FRIEND THOMAS IS ALLERGIC TO SEAFOOD AND NUTS. HE OUTGREW HIS BEEF ALLERGY.

SUMMER CAMP

Three summers ago, I went to a weeklong summer camp. This was a huge step for me. A big help was that my best friend since fourth grade, Thomas, was going, too. It just so happens that he's allergic to nuts and shellfish.

It was our first time being on our own for a week, and I knew we'd look out for each other. We visited the camp's chef a few weeks beforehand to make sure it was even possible for us to go. Of course, they had had campers with allergies before. At every meal, I asked the chef what he was making, and he would tell me if I could have it or not.

I had to be very careful about what I ate. I packed a lot of my own snacks and candy. I remember Thomas

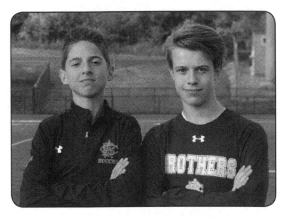

MY BEST FRIEND THOMAS
WHO HAS FOOD ALLERGIES TOO

came in with bags of cereal and tons of stuff because he thought he wasn't going to be able to eat anything.

On the other hand, my other friend James was also at camp with us. He's not allergic to anything, and he was a jokester back then. He would get so hyper just from eating one AirHead!

In this case, he came with three boxes of AirHeads, and each box had 100 of the taffy-like candies in it. Every night we could visit the canteen and pick out two pieces of candy. They had EVERYTHING from ice cream to Skittles, to Hershey's bars, to Chex Mix, to soda. It was crazy! There wasn't much I could eat there, so I was grateful James brought all of those AirHeads!

A SILVER LINING

The one good thing about having food allergies is that reading labels has made me a healthy eater. I can't have most store-bought desserts, cakes, cupcakes, or muffins. I don't think most people realize all the unhealthy garbage that's in food like frosting. Some processed frosting even has beef fat in it! After I read that, I will never look at frosting the same way again.

I love to eat salads because they are very healthy and mostly contain no cheese. In fact, my whole family eats healthier, I think, because we have to think about food so much.

YOUR LIFE WITH ALLERGIES:

- How do you manage your food allergies at school?

- Are all of your friends, coaches, and teachers trained to use auto-injectors?

- What's your biggest worry about allergies at school?

- How do you handle eating at restaurants? Are you comfortable ordering and explaining your allergics to your server? What are your best and worst experiences at a restaurant?

- How do you manage your food allergies when traveling? If you travel to a foreign country, how do you communicate with the people cooking and serving your food about the ingredients in it?

- How do your food allergies impact your social life? In which situations do you feel most uncomfortable?

- Have there been activities you haven't participated in because of your food allergies? What could've made these situations safer?

DECIPHERING FOOD LABELS

I have a friend who is allergic to peanuts, who didn't know how to read food labels. Before he ate a food, instead of looking at the label, he would look at the food and smell it to see if it contained peanuts. No joke! Obviously, this was very dumb, because you can't always see or smell peanuts in a food.

Interpreting food labels is a crucial skill if you have food allergies. The rule of thumb is that you MUST read the label before you eat anything! If you can't read a food label, you become vulnerable to having an allergic reaction.

The Food Allergen Labeling and Consumer Protection Act (FALCPA) is the federal law governing how ingredients are represented on packaged foods in the U.S. This act is effective for all foods, vitamins, dietary supplements, infant foods, and more. The FALCPA covers the eight most common allergens: peanuts, tree nuts, dairy, wheat, fish, soy, egg, and shellfish. Unfortunately, if you are allergic to a food not on this list, such as sesame seeds, you may have to dig deeper (i.e., call the manufacturer) to find out if a food is safe to east.

FALCPA dictates how food companies have to label their ingredients. Because this is a federal law, it applies to every state. The law gives manufacturers a choice on declaring allergens in their products. The allergen can be listed in an ingredient list OR in a separate "contains" statement.

Looking at a food label can be overwhelming because processed foods often have twenty or so ingredients listed in tiny print! If there is not a "contains" statement, unfortunately, you need to read the entire ingredient list and hunt down your allergens.

A "contains" label will appear at the bottom of the ingredient list and say in bold letters something like, **"Contains: Wheat and Soy."** Instead of having to read every ingredient, you can see quickly that the food contains wheat and soy. This is obviously much easier to deal with.

But remember: *if there is no "contains" statement, it does not mean the food doesn't contain allergens!* It could simply mean that the manufacturer chose to declare the allergen in the ingredient list instead.

Some nutrition labels may say something at the very bottom like: "Made on shared equipment that also processes wheat and soy." This means that product was manufactured on a piece of equipment that also is used for food containing wheat and soy. It is assumed the equipment would be cleaned in between products, but there is a risk of residue remaining on the machine. Whether or not you eat a product with this type of warning is a decision you should make with your allergist.

You will also come across statements that say: "May contain wheat and soy." Similar to the previous warning, this "May contain" is the manufacturer letting you know the product might contain these allergens. Manufacturers aren't required to put this on their labels; it's voluntary. Again, discuss this warning with your doctor. In my case, I never eat anything that "may contain" my allergen. Too risky for me!

Yet another phrase you might see is: "Made in a facility that also produces products with peanuts." In this case, the manufacturer makes something in their facility with nuts, although there shouldn't be nuts in that particular product. However, the risk exists that a mistake could occur and a nut might end up in that product.

Even with FALCPA, mistakes are made frequently and foods are recalled. A recall is when a manufacturer alerts the public and the FDA that a food contains ingredients NOT listed on their label. If a manufacturer's recall wasn't announced, it could result in a fatal allergic reaction in one of their consumers.

If you ever feel like you are having an allergic reaction from a product that doesn't have your allergen on the label, call the manufacturer because it might not be your imagination. Also, sign up for FARE's recall alert emails so that you'll be in the know before you take a bite.

The safest foods are those that are made in a facility not containing your allergen. Manufacturers will often put these safety practices on their packages. For instance, you might have seen labels that read: "Made in a peanut-free facility." Enjoy Life Foods are labeled "Allergy Friendly" because they are free from gluten and fourteen common allergens.

Another point about food labels is knowing how to identify your allergen. For example, milk is not always labeled as milk. I had to learn that "whey" and "casein" are milk ingredients I'm allergic to. This is something you should also ask your doctor about.

The last point I want to make about food labels is that they can change. One granola bar I had eaten for a long time suddenly had milk listed on the label. This is normal because manufacturers are continually trying to improve their products and recipes can change. Don't get lazy when reading food labels.

I heard about a teen recently who had a fatal allergic reaction. She ate a packaged cookie she had eaten before but didn't realize the company now made a version with peanut butter. It's imperative to always check labels even on something you've eaten in the past.

WHAT ARE YOUR RULES WHEN READING A FOOD LABEL?

- To practice, go to the pantry and pick out two foods: one you know is safe for you to eat and one that isn't. Do the nutrition labels have "Contain" statements? Do you see your allergen on the ingredients list?

- Visit www.foodallergy.org/common-allergens /allergy-alerts and sign up for FARE's emailed recall alerts.

MY SUPPORT SQUAD

If you know someone with food allergies, supporting them in daily life is crucial. My personal support squad includes my parents, brothers, grandparents, cousins, aunts, uncles, teachers, babysitters, and my allergist. These are the people in my life who not only watch out for the foods I eat, but who also try to understand the stress I sometimes feel. They help me feel safer and more like a normal teenager who just happens to have food allergies.

First and foremost, my support squad is aware of my allergies, and they help me look out for dangerous foods. They all know how to use my auto-injector. Even though the auto-injector has instructions on it, it's a good idea to review them occasionally.

My mom is very helpful to me when it comes to cooking. She has many allergen-free cookbooks with great recipe ideas. She and my dad are careful about choosing restaurants for family dinners.

When I visit my grandparents or my aunts, they make a lot of effort to stock up on safe foods for me, which means a lot. Of course, sometimes mistakes happen.

Every time we go to Texas, my aunt makes fun pancakes in the shape of the state, along with ones in the shape of a ten-gallon hat and a cowboy boot. Once, she accidentally put dairy milk in the batter. She was so concerned about having the non-dairy margarine on the table, she didn't even think about the milk. I felt bad for her because I know she didn't mean it.

My grandfather loves ice cream, and he's notorious for ordering flavors with nuts when my brother and I go out for ice cream with him. Once, at Ted Drewes, a famous custard shop in St. Louis, we didn't keep an eye on him, and he ordered butter pecan.

"Dad, did you get something with nuts?!" my mom asked.

"Oh, shoot," he replied.

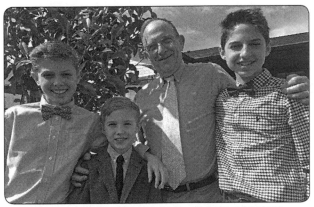

WITH MY BROTHERS AND GRANDFATHER

Even though it was raining, my mom didn't let him get in the car! We love to tease him about this story. Sometimes my grandpa can be in a different world, but I love him so much and I know he'd never intentionally put me in danger.

My friends are very supportive as well. While my best friend has allergies, my other friends do not. It's important for all of my friends to know about my allergies. If you're new to allergies and worried about telling your friends, remember that this is not something to be shy about. For example, if someone has a peanut butter sandwich at lunch, they will tell me and sit a few seats down from me. I feel really good when this happens because I know my friends look out for me.

Fortunately, no one has ever bullied me about my allergies. Now that I'm in high school, I spend more time with my friends in social situations. It's important to have friends I can trust who understand.

My school is also a source of support for me. As I've mentioned, I meet with the cafeteria staff before school begins to review lunch options. I make sure my teachers and the school nurse are aware of my allergies as well.

In addition to my personal support team, there is also a national food allergy community that I am part of. My family is a member of FARE, the Food Allergy Research and Education organization, whose mission it is to advocate for people with food allergies. FARE played a big role in passing the School Access to Emergency Epinephrine Act in 2013, which helped schools across the U.S. stock epinephrine in their clinics and nurses' offices. FARE's website, which has helped me in the past, is filled with allergy facts and news. This is very important to me because I can check out the site or their Twitter account and know what's going on in the food allergy world.

My mom and I also receive FARE's alerts about recalls and contaminated foods, which I mentioned in the last chapter. The U.S. Food and Drug Administration (the FDA) is in charge of keeping our food safe. They are the ones that issue recalls or warnings about food safety. Sometimes a food accidentally contains an allergen, and FARE is great about letting the food allergy community know.

Every year I try to go to one of FARE's allergy awareness walks. It's an opportunity for me to be with other kids who have allergies and to raise money for research. There are fun activities and samples of new allergen-free products to try.

This year, I went to FARE's annual Teen Summit. I learned a lot from other teens and about new research being done.

Unlike other kids, those of us with food allergies have to be responsible for our own personal safety at a young age. Studies show that kids with food allergies have higher anxiety, which makes sense to me—we always have something to worry about. We worry about what ingredients are in foods and about accidentally eating an allergen. It's extra stress other kids don't have, and stress is unhealthy.

It's important to talk to someone if you feel worried or stressed. Think about talking to your support squad, and don't be afraid to talk to a counselor or therapist. I've done that before. They can really help because they are trained to guide you through your struggles.

Knowing you have a group of people on your side makes living with food allergies a lot easier. I've created a worksheet to help you get started!

SUPPORT SQUAD WORKSHEET

Having a support squad that is aware of your condition and knows how to treat it is one of the keys to a happy and less stressful life with food allergies. To assemble your own support squad, start by answering the following questions:

Which family member(s) always have your back?

_____

_____

Of those family members, which ones spend the most time with you?

_____

Are there any teachers or coaches you feel comfortable talking to?

_____

_____

Who prepares food for you or buys your groceries? _____

_____

Who is the friend you spend the most time with and who knows you very well?

_____

Name all the people you know who have food allergies. _____

_____

_____

Which doctor or nurse do you feel most comfortable talking to about your allergies?

_____

_____

If you're feeling anxious, is there a counselor that you could discuss your allergies with?

_____

Now, take a look at all the people you identified. A good support squad will ideally include a combination of the following:

- individuals who live, cook, and eat with you
- a friend you spend a lot of time with
- a medical professional
- someone from school
- someone you can call anytime to talk about anything related to your allergies

Go back over the list of people. Can you circle the names of the people who would be the biggest help to you? Write their names here:

_____

_____

_____

_____

_____

Congratulations! You've just created a potential support squad! Review this list with a parent or trusted adult, and then plan to tell these people the role you'd like them to play in helping you manage your allergies.

TEEN TALK

RISKY BUSINESS

Being a teenager isn't always easy, and if you have food allergies, it's one more thing to deal with. In fact, it's the riskiest time in your life to have food allergies.

Teens and young adults have a higher risk of having a **fatal** *allergic reaction.*

Why?

1. **Denying symptoms.** Teens sometimes downplay or deny their symptoms, so the reaction gets out of control.

2. **Medication not available.** Many teens don't carry their medication with them. They might assume, for example, they won't eat any nuts at a party, so they don't take their auto-injector with them.

3. **Delay in using auto-injector.** If they do have it with them, teens often wait too long to use their auto-injector.

4. **Peer pressure.** Teens want to fit in and be like everyone else. They might refuse to carry medication with them because they don't want to draw attention to themselves. Or they might think it's embarrassing to tell people about their allergies.

5. **New social scene.** The teen years are when kids start having their own social lives—going out with friends to sports games, movies, parties, restaurants, etc. Even though teens don't want to speak up about allergies, it's exactly the time when they MUST speak up.

6. **Brain development.** During puberty, the brain is still developing. Teenagers are more likely to do dumb stuff like driving too fast, taking drugs, drinking, and smoking.

The question is, why do teenagers take more risks than adults?

There's been a lot of research lately about teenage brains. Psychologist Dr. Laurence Steinberg is quoted in *Allergic Living* as claiming that the brain is not growing during these years as much as it's being reorganized. "All of the changes [in the brain] take place in the regions that regulate the experience of pleasure, the ways we in which we view and think about other people, and our ability to exercise self-control."[7] This means that the teenage brain is not always able to evaluate risks or to make good decisions. On top of that, having food allergies is ANOTHER risk we must be careful about.

Any one of these circumstances increases a teen's risk.

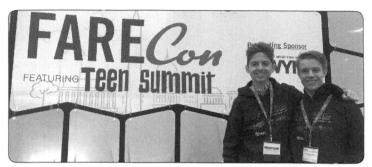

THOMAS AND I MET LOTS OF OTHER TEENS AT FARE'S 2018 FOOD ALLERGY CONFERENCE.

ALLERGY ANXIETIES

As I mentioned before, teenagers with food allergies also have a higher rate of anxiety and depression. Teenagers can also be more stressed or depressed because they are worried about their allergies. A recent study in Canada found that "children with food allerg[ies] were about twice as likely to experience mental health problems than young people without food allergies."[8]

I'm not surprised by this statistic. It's logical that kids with food allergies have more anxiety. We eat three meals a day plus snacks, and for a person with food allergies, that's at least three to five times per day they have to think about their allergies. For the average person, going out to eat or to a party or sitting down to eat lunch at school is a relaxing, social time. When you have food allergies, these situations can cause anxiety, not just from fear of a reaction but from worrying about what others think about you.

My food allergies make me feel stressed at times. I can feel nervous or anxious around new friends and situations. Sometimes, you don't even know how the stress impacts you. In the past, I've met with a psychologist about my anxiety. I'm not embarrassed about that at all. Just like we go to a dentist for our teeth or a doctor when we have the flu, we sometimes need a doctor for our mental health. Many schools have psychologists on staff, which can be a good place to start talking about your anxiety. Alternatively, your allergist or general doctor can help find you a good psychologist.

I found it helpful to talk with my psychologist, especially because she taught me a few techniques for handling stressful situations. One that really works for me is a breathing exercise. I also learned with her help my stress level goes down when I feel in control and prepared, which is part of the reason why I bring my auto-injector with me everywhere.

Everyone will experience stress at some point in their life, so figure out what coping strategies work for you sooner rather than later!

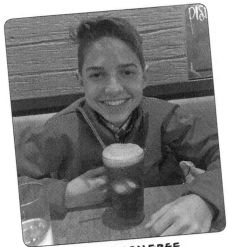

ALLERGEN FREE
ROOT BEER FLOAT

A BALANCING ACT

While all of this sounds overwhelming, the way I keep things in perspective is the concept of balance. What I mean by that is balancing being cautious with *living*. Even with allergies, it is possible to enjoy food, and it's important for food-allergic kids to feel they can do "normal" things like everyone else. Along with your allergist and your parents, you will need to find your comfort level and set safe boundaries.

For example, if you are allergic to nuts, can you eat foods that are labeled as "made on shared equipment," "may contain nuts," or "made in a facility that also makes nut products"? Can you feel safe at a restaurant? Are there certain restaurants to avoid?

Despite my dairy allergy, I love going out to eat frozen yogurt. There are usually one or two non-dairy flavors to choose from. However, I don't get my toppings from the toppings bar. The place I go serves my toppings directly from the original containers behind the counter. This way I avoid any potential cross-contamination, and I feel both comfortable and careful.

On the other hand, a friend of mine who is also allergic to nuts will not go to these types of places. Since there are nuts in some of the flavors, he doesn't trust that the machines get cleaned well enough. He's not comfortable, so he doesn't take the risk. These are the types of decisions a kid with food allergies has to face every day.

Here are my action items for teens to decrease their food allergy risk and anxiety:

1. **Speak up.** Tell your friends that you have food allergies, so they can make sure not to eat your allergen when they are around you. When you're a teen, you may go to parties and go out a lot with your friends. You have the right to feel comfortable when you're with them, and if they know you have food allergies and they know how to use an auto-injector, you may be able to relax more easily. It's also important

to speak up about your allergies when you start to date. Kissing someone who has eaten something you're allergic to could give you a reaction.

2. **Make sure you carry your medication every-where you go.** Have a plan! Where will you keep your auto-injector? In a purse? A fanny pack? You need to have a procedure, so you never forget it. Before I go anywhere, I decide what I will carry it in: a backpack, cross-body messenger bag, a carrier on my waist, etc. I want to look like everyone else, but safety is priority. I also wear a medical bracelet.

3. **Work with your parents on hypothetical allergy scenarios.** Practice decision-making so that when you're living on your own (i.e., at camp, in college, or after high school grad-uation) you know what to do. Even though parents want to protect you, they should help you develop independence because soon you will not be in their protective environment.

4. **Get connected with the food allergy com-munity.** There are many online resources (websites, blogs) specifically for teens with food allergies. There is a Canadian website, www.whyriskit.ca, that provides good infor-mation for teens. You might even want to

attend an event such as FARE's annual Teen Summit where you can go and socialize with other teens who have food allergies.

5. **Don't be afraid to talk to a professional if you feel anxious about your allergies.** Talking with a counselor doesn't show weakness, so don't be afraid to do it. If cost is a concern, there might be a counselor at your school.

WHAT ABOUT YOU?

- What do you carry your auto-injector in? Is it visible to others?

- Do your friends know about your allergies? Do they know what to do if you have a reaction?

- Do you ever feel embarrassed when talking about your food allergies?

- How do your allergies impact your stress level?

- Complete the following sentences:

  I feel most scared about my allergies when
  _____ .

  I feel safest when eating _____ .

LOOKING AHEAD

Now that I'm fifteen, my hope to outgrow my food allergies is statistically smaller. However, I'm optimistic about some of the new therapies being developed and the trials going on. My dream is to one day drink a medicine that will cure my allergies.

Another dream is that epinephrine could be a small pill that's easier for people to take. I recently read about some guys who are trying to build an auto-injector into a phone case, which sounds super cool.

I also would like to see pharmaceutical companies giving free auto-injectors to the poor and to people who can't afford them. It is a life-saving drug, and it does not need to have its price bumped up like an expensive new car or "must-have" designer clothes.

Restaurant menus are improving, and I hope more will label menu items peanut-free, soy-free, dairy-free, etc. Not only does it make it easier for people with allergies and the staff who have to field their questions, but it may attract more customers to those restaurants.

There is more awareness of food allergies now than ever before, but there is still more education to be shared. For example, people I meet almost always assume my dairy allergy is an intolerance. Most people know how deadly a peanut allergy can be, but we need more education about the severity of other allergies.

One of my main fears is going to someone's house or to a party and asking them for something to eat and them telling me the wrong ingredients. I think about this more as I get older and go to places on my own. I am transitioning from my parents being the leaders of my support team to taking that role myself.

In fact, this summer we went to Argentina again for a month, and I wanted stay with a host family. This meant I would have someone who doesn't speak English cooking dinner for me in their home every night. The Spanish school found a woman who was willing to take on the challenge of hosting me. Before I arrived, we had to explain my allergies, especially about my dairy allergy, because she, like most people, thought I was lactose intolerant. I also showed her when I arrived how to use my auto-injector.

Every night before dinner, we reviewed all the ingredients she used. There was only one night where we figured out before dinner that she had used a sauce packet that said "may contain nuts."

I had to be super careful, but I had a great time and she was an awesome cook!

APPENDICES

WORDS TO KNOW

Allergy: A damaging immune response by the body to a substance, especially pollen, fur, a particular food, or dust, to which it has become hypersensitive.

Anaphylaxis: An acute allergic reaction to an antigen (e.g., a bee sting) to which the body has become hypersensitive.

Antihistamine: A drug or other compound that inhibits the physiological effects of histamine, used especially in the treatment of allergies.

Auto-injector: An pre-filled injection containing epinephrine, a chemical that narrows blood vessels and opens airways in the lungs. These effects can reverse severe low blood pressure, wheezing, severe skin itching, hives, and other symptoms of an allergic reaction.

Cross-contamination: The process by which bacteria or other microorganisms are unintentionally transferred from one substance or object to another, with harmful effect(s).

Histamine: A compound that is released by cells in response to injury and in allergic and inflammatory reactions, causing contraction of smooth muscle and dilation of capillaries

Immune System: A body system made up of a network of cells, tissues, and organs that work together to protect the body. The important cells involved are white blood cells, which seek out and destroy disease-causing organisms or substances.

Intolerance: An inability to eat a food or take a drug without adverse effects.

Definitions from Google Dictionary. Google Search. Google. Web. 3 Jul. 2018.

JUST DIAGNOSED WITH A FOOD ALLERGY?

Olivier's Plan of Action!

If you were recently diagnosed with a food allergy, you may be confused on what to do next. Let me help you out with the following step-by-step suggestions.

1. **See an Allergist.** Most likely you had a reaction and have seen your general practitioner or family doctor, who may have given you a prescription for an auto-injector. If possible, I highly recommend seeing a board-certified allergist in addition to seeing your regular doctor.

2. **Recognize a Reaction.** Learn how to recognize an allergic reaction in yourself. Reactions are different for everyone, so you need to be aware of what happens in your body so you can identify the reaction immediately.

3. **Educate Those around You.** Sit down with your family, friends, coaches, and others to tell them what to do in case of a reaction. Show them how to use the auto-injector. To help, the next section of this book is a page you can give directly to your friends.

4. **Create Your Support Squad.** You will find a helpful worksheet to form your own support squad on page 69 of this book.

5. **School Preparation.** Talk to your school about their food policies and their rules about carrying your auto-injector. Make sure the school nurse has an auto-injector and that all of the staff has been trained to use one. Your parents can help with this because you will probably need an allergy action plan on file at school as well. In addition, there is something called a 504 Plan that you might need. This is a plan that helps kids with legally recognized disabilities – including food allergies – get access to the resources they need to succeed academically. These and other emergency care plans can be written up so your teachers have procedures in place to keep students with allergies safe at school.

6. **Get Connected.** Check out the Food Allergy Research & Education website (**www. foodallergy.org**) and sign up for their recall alerts. The site has many useful resources including information on support groups.

   One way I've decided to get connected is by starting a club at my school. With the support of my principal, I started the FAAB Club last year, which stands for Food Allergy &

Awareness Brothers. ("Brothers" because my
school is Christian Brothers Academy.) We had
a couple of events, including an auto-injector
training session. We hope to have more events
this year to expand awareness, not just of
food allergies but of other food-related issues
as well. My goal is to put a template together
other teens can take to their schools.

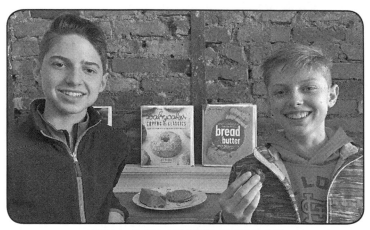

ERIN MCKENNA'S BAKERY IN NYC
IS ALLERGY FRIENDLY

7. **Go Shopping! Explore your local grocery store
and check out which foods are safe for you.**
Be open to trying new things; you might be
surprised by how much you like them. Many
grocery stores have cards that allow you to
request new products so keep that in mind

if there's something you'd like your store to carry. You may also consider buying a medical bracelet and an auto-injector carrier. It's nice to be able to wear something with your name, contact information, and medication all together. (For more specifics, check out my resources page.)

8. **Have a Good Attitude.** Finally, try to be positive about your new situation even if you feel stressed. If you do feel anxious, don't be afraid to talk to somebody about it. There is probably even a counselor at your school to help with this. Remember that it's okay to feel stressed. After all, having a food allergy is a big deal.

   Also, have a good attitude towards others around you. Don't *expect* people to accommodate your allergies. If you're going to someone's house, offer to bring your own food, for example.

FOR YOUR FRIENDS...

Are you uncomfortable talking to your friends about your allergies? Don't be. Think about it from their point of view. They care about you and want to be supportive.

Last year, I read an article written by the friends of someone who had had an allergic reaction when they were all together. However, the teen with the allergies had never fully explained to his friends what he was allergic to and what needed to happen if he ingested his allergen. When he had a bad reaction, his friends felt helpless. They all wished their friend had spoken up ahead of time, before it was too late.[9]

Talking to your friends is for their sake as well. (And honestly, if your friends aren't supportive and don't take your allergies seriously, maybe it's time for new friends.)

The next page can be given directly to your friends. You can also text your friends a link to the information. The link can be found at:

WhenEveryBiteMatters.com

KNOW SOMEONE WITH FOOD ALLERGIES?

Here's What You Can Do!

We all know someone with a food allergy. Allergies are different for everyone, so what's the best way to be a good friend? Here are a few ideas:

1. **Listen and understand.** When your friend tells you about their allergy, make sure to listen and ask questions. You must understand how severe the allergy is. If he/she is allergic to nuts and you bring a peanut butter sandwich for lunch, for example, make sure you don't sit with your friend. Depending on the severity of the allergy, you may need to wash your hands after lunch and before you can touch them again (e.g., for a handshake, game of tag).

2. **Know how to recognize a reaction.** Reactions can vary greatly from person to person. Talk to your friend about what happens to them when they have a reaction so you can recognize it if you are with them.

3. **Know where the auto-injector is located and how to use it.** Most auto-injectors have instructions on them, but if someone is having a reaction, every second counts. Your friend might have a trainer you can practice with. Of

course, you will also need to know where your friend's medication is, so make sure they tell you where they tend to keep it.

4. **Look out for your friend.** Look out for your friend when you guys are doing an activity or going to a party together. You should also support your friend if they need to carry medicine. Remind them to have it with them and let them know they don't look weird!

5. **Support your friend if they experience peer pressure.** Sometimes even well-meaning people will try to pressure allergy sufferers into risky situations. For example, if all your friends want to go to a Thai restaurant and your friend with food allergies can't eat there because of all of the nuts, try to get your friends to eat somewhere else. Keep in mind a list of safe places your friend can enjoy. Also, try to stop anyone who might be teasing your friend about their allergies. People who joke about allergies don't understand how serious they are.

6. **"Close friends."** If you are the boyfriend or girlfriend of someone with allergies, you're going to have understand how to be safe when holding their hands and kissing them. If you drink a milkshake and then kiss someone

who's allergic to milk, they'll have a reaction. Of course it feels embarrassing to talk about, but it's necessary to set the ground rules ahead of time!

7. **Want more info? If you want to educate yourself about allergies, there are great resources online.** A great place to start is www.foodallergy.org.

PARENT TO PARENT

My food allergies, and my brother's, affect our whole family. I've asked my mom to share her perspective, which might be helpful to your parents:

Having children with food allergies certainly increases the complexity of the already challenging task of parenting! Since Olivier was diagnosed when he was four months old, this is the only world my husband Greg and I have known as parents. It was a shock initially, and we had no idea what this journey would entail.

For any parents of food-allergic kids, especially those who have been recently diagnosed, I know it's overwhelming, stressful, and depressing, but *you are not alone. You can do this.*

Parenting involves a lot of risk management. Think of parenting a food-allergic child as taking that to a higher level.

Olivier and Mathias' food allergies steer a lot of what we do as a family: where we eat out, where we vacation, how we cook at home, etc. We enjoy entertaining a lot at home, but we also do it because it's safer for the boys. One of the trickiest things socially is when people invite us over for dinner. (The brave ones, that is, because many are too afraid.) People mean well and offer to cook safe food for the boys, but how can you tell someone, "Hey, we can't trust you. We can't trust your handling of cross-contamination"? What's more, a host shouldn't be expected to know the ins and outs of cooking for the boys, so these situations are tricky.

It can be frustrating at times. While most people have an understanding of a peanut allergy, many do not realize Olivier's milk allergy is just as life-threatening. Patience is required!

My strategy in many allergy situations is to be kind and accommodating but still firm. I never *expect* anyone to accommodate the boys' allergies. Offering to bring food or dessert takes the burden off of the other person.

Life with the boys significantly improved when they learned to speak. Prior to that, I only knew they were having a reaction by seeing a physical symptom. It's a scary way to live, especially because their allergies were evolving.

We've made our share of mistakes along the way. No one can be perfect. A parenting book I had said to introduce scrambled eggs at around nine months. No one had told me Olivier might be allergic to more than milk, so of course one night I gave him eggs and he was suddenly covered with hives. We had just moved and were living in a hotel. I hadn't even met our new pediatrician yet and had to make an emergency call to him. He must have thought I was crazy!

Then there was the time at the crowded local ice cream stand. Greg and I were socializing when Mathias ran up to us, "Can I get the trash can sundae?" Sure, we said, having no idea until a few minutes later it was covered in peanut sauce.

My husband and I (and the boys) had a huge fear of using the epinephrine auto-injector at first. In hindsight, there were a few times we should have given it but didn't because we were scared, and their reaction seemed to be controlled with Benadryl. We now realize those situations could have easily turned out differently because airways can close up in seconds.

Our allergist in Connecticut used to say to me, "No one dies from an EpiPen." Still, the thought of using an auto-injector is frightening. I think this is actually less about the auto-injector and more about the intensity of what's probably taking place when you need it.

My husband recommends not thinking of **if** you will use the auto-injector but **when**. Depending on your child's situation, in all the thousands of times they consume food, it's likely there will be a mistake made.

Prepare for it. Talk with your allergist to understand exactly when epinephrine should be used. Stick to these instructions and don't second-guess yourself in the moment. Practice using the auto-injector and reassuring your child. Yes, the first time you need to use it will be an overwhelming situation, but it is the best and only way to stop a reaction quickly.

The first time we needed to use it was a traumatic situation, but it was also followed by the relief that the auto-injector itself wasn't so bad. We all now understand delaying use of the auto-injector is what is dangerous. Epi first, epi fast.

From an early age, we've taught both boys to speak up and to communicate about their allergies. It's important to guide them toward independence and self-advocacy, especially with regards to carrying their medication with them. I still usually have a back-up, but grabbing their packs must become instinctive.

A big challenge I find with parenting the boys is teaching them not to trust. Mathias is more impulsive and open by nature. For example, if cookies are being served after church, he'll ask if they contain nuts. If he's told no, he thinks it's safe. I've had to drill into him that the volunteer has no idea, and without a clear label, he cannot eat anything. "No label, no eat." This has been my mantra with him. It was difficult for him to learn that even though people try to be nice, what they say can't be trusted in terms of his allergies. And he's a kid! He wants the cookie! Thankfully, he gets it now.

I'm not going to lie, as they enter these teenage years, it doesn't get better. Now, they self-carry their medication at school, they are away from me more, and have to take on more of the responsibility for their allergies themselves.

Every time we leave the house, I ask, "Do you have your EpiPen?" I constantly think in my head: "Did I remind him not to eat the cake?" "What if someone gives him a cookie?" etc.

Now we have other issues to discuss such as girl-friends, alcohol, and drugs. We've started talking about how when people with food allergies are impaired by a substance they may forget and eat something they're allergic to, or they might forget their medication or not be able to use it properly.

While it's a similar message any parent might communicate to their teen, having food allergies adds complications.

As I write this, we are in Argentina, where the boys are studying Spanish. Olivier very much wanted to stay with a host family. Again, this presented a much more complicated situation with his allergies. How could I let a stranger in a foreign country cook dinner for him every night? Well, we did it! We explained the allergies ahead of time, and Olivier's conscientiousness combined with his hostess's desire to have him turned out successfully. (Plus, I'm staying exactly one block away, and I FaceTime him every night after dinner and remind him to check before he eats!) It was more stressful for me as his mother, but having this opportunity has increased Olivier's confidence.

On the positive side of food allergies are all the changes I've seen over the past fifteen years. Food allergy awareness has greatly increased. Awareness saves lives. I heard a doctor speak recently who said the world food allergy sufferers live in is divided into two groups: people who get it and people who don't.

There are significantly more allergen-friendly foods available now, and technology allows both the quick dissemination of information (such as product recalls) as well as many platforms for support (blogs, social groups).

We can NEVER let our guard down around food. My heart sinks when I read about fatal allergic reactions. The truth is the boys' allergies are a constant worry and I hate they have them. However, our lives are richly blessed in many ways, and the boys rarely complain. The attitude Olivier conveys in this book is how we live as a family. Yes, the allergies stink, and we have to deal with them by living cautiously, but we still live life to the fullest.

—ALISON DELDICQUE

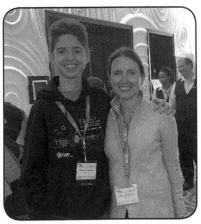

MOM AND I AT THE FARECON
TEEN SUMMIT ON FOOD ALLERGIES.

NOTES

1. Food Allergy Research & Education. What is a Food Allergy? www.foodallergy.org/life-with-food-allergies/food-allergy-101/what-is-a-food-allergy. Accessed 20 Jun 2018.

2. FAIR Health, Inc. Claim Lines with Diagnoses of Anaphylactic Food Reactions Climbed 377 Percent from 2007 to 2016. www.fairhealth.org/press-release/claim-lines-with-diagnoses-of-anaphylactic-food-reactions-climbed-377-percent-from-2007-to-2016; version 08.2017. Accessed 20 Jun 2018.

3. Food Allergy Research & Education. Facts and Statistics. www.foodallergy.org/life-with-food-allergies/food-allergy-101/facts-and-statistics. Accessed 20 Jun 2018.

4. Branum AM, Lukacs SL. Food allergy among U.S. children: trends in prevalence and hospitalizations. *NCHS Data Brief.* 2008;10:1-8.

5. Decker WW, Campbell RL, Manivannan V, et al. The etiology and incidence of anaphylaxis in Rochester, Minnesota: a report from the Rochester Epidemiology Project. *J Allergy Clin Immunol.* 2008;122(6):1161-1165.

6. Skin patch to treat peanut allergy shows benefit in children. *National Institutes of Health.* 26 Oct. 2016. www.nih.gov/news-events/news-releases/skin-patch-treat-peanut-allergy-shows-benefit-children. Accessed 5 Sep. 2018.

7. Hewett, H. Food Allergy Meets the Teenage Brain. *Allergic Living.* 23 Nov. 2015. www.allergicliving. com/2015/11/23/food-allergy-meets-the-teenage-brain.

8. Teenagers With Food Allergies Face Higher Rates of Depression, Anxiety, Study Finds. *Allergic Living.* 21 Jan. 2016. www.allergicliving.com/2016/01/21/teenagers-with-food-allergies-face-higher-rates-of-depression-anxiety-study-finds/.

9. Smith, N. "Simon Katz's Friends on a Food Allergy Tragedy: What We Wish We'd Known." *Allergic Living.* 19 Apr 2017. www.allergicliving.com/2017/04/19/simon-katzs-friends-on-a-food-allergy-tragedy-what-we-wish-wed-known/. Accessed 9 Aug 2018.

COOL RESOURCES
TO CHECK OUT!

INFORMATION

Allergic Living Magazine
www.allergicliving.com

This site is great, but I also receive the magazine. It has informative articles, and even the ads are good because they are often for new products and allergen-free foods.

Auvi-Q
www.auvi-q.com

The Auvi-Q is a type of auto-injector, and their site contains useful information about the product. The Auvi-Q comes in a square shape that can fit in your pants pocket. It comes with audio instructions that walk you through the use of the product with the press of a button.

EpiPen
www.epipen.com

If you have a prescription for an EpiPen, you can register it on this site. The company will send you a free pouch to carry your EpiPen in and will also let you know when your auto-injector expires.

FAACT (Food Allergy & Anaphylaxis Connection Team)
www.foodallergyawareness.org

This site has a lot of great information that's helpful if you are newly diagnosed. They also have pages about summer camps for children and teenagers with food allergies.

FARE (Food Allergy Research & Education)
www.foodallergy.org

I think FARE is the best allergy website there is. They list lots of facts and news about allergies that really help me out a lot. They post the newest studies about food allergies and also send out alerts on food recalls.

This link takes you directly to the page on food allergy laws and regulations: **www.foodallergy.org/life-with-food-allergies/ newly-diagnosed/laws-and-regulations**.

Kids with Food Allergies
www.kidswithfoodallergies.org

Another reliable site with a lot of information on food allergies—and many recipes, too!

Medline Plus
www.medlineplus.gov

Published by the National Institutes of Health, this is a reliable source for medical information on a wide range of topics, including food allergies.

Why Risk It?
www.whyriskit.ca

This Canadian site is especially for teens trying to balance their food allergies with living a normal life!

COOL MERCHANDISE

There are many places online to buy charms, sticker or patches that say "EpiPen Inside." This is a great idea to put on your backpack so people know where to find your medication.

As for what to carry your medication in, this is really a personal choice. (It's easier for girls who carry purses!) There are many designs available. My brother, for instance, uses a runner's belt that expands enough to fit everything in. His is a SPIbelt we got on Amazon.

Sometimes I use a travel pouch designed to carry a passport under your shirt. There are times when having this around my waist is the best way to go. Mostly, though, I carry my medication inside a backpack. Just keep an eye on the temperature, especially if you're outside on a hot or cold day, because this can impact the effectiveness of the epinephrine.

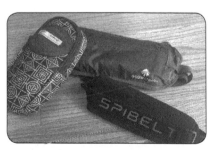
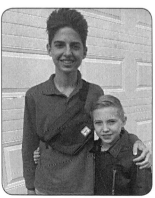

THESE ARE SOME OF THE DIFFERENT CASES I USE TO CARRY MY AUTO-INJECTORS.

Allergy Apparel
www.allergyapparel.com

Allergy Apparel has very fancy auto-injector carriers and medical ID bracelets. They have a large selection to choose from, and their designs are sweet! The bracelets here are very stylish.

American Medical ID
www.americanmedical-id.com

To help medical personnel know my allergy information quickly, I wear a stainless steel bracelet I bought from this site. It's great quality, somewhat stylish, but still looks like a medical bracelet.

Chef Cards
safefare.org/chefcard

Follow this link to print cards you can give to a restaurant with all your allergies listed in many different languages. There are other sites where you can buy these already laminated and premade. However, here you can print it for free!

Lauren's Hope
www.laurenshope.com

Lauren's Hope has really cool creative bracelets and necklaces for your food allergy ID. They have great designs for boys and girls.

LegBuddy
www.omaxcare.com/legbuddy

A girl I met at camp this summer carried her auto-injector in this pouch strapped to her leg. She said it worked great for her.

FAVORITE FOOD SITES

Amy's Kitchen
www.amys.com

I like Amy's non-dairy breakfast burritos, pizza, and many of the soups. They make a lot of allergen-friendly food.

Daiya
www.daiyafoods.com

Daiya cheese is the main reason why I don't hate my life with food allergies! Their cheese is amazing! Now they make macaroni and cheese and pizzas, too.

Earth Balance
www.earthbalancenatural.com

Earth Balance makes the "butter" I eat, and we use their products for baking. They make great snacks, like their aged "white cheddar" popcorn, too.

Enjoy Life
enjoylifefoods.com

Enjoy Life has many food products that are dairy-free, nut-free, gluten-free, and so much more! My personal favorites are their cookies and granola bars.

Food Allergy Mama Baking Book

Available at Amazon.com, Kelly Rudnicki's book has the best recipes for allergen-free cooking. I cook a lot from this baking cookbook because the recipes are easy and delicious!

free2b Foods
https://free2bfoods.com/

free2b has many yummy snacks free from 12 top allergens. Their dark chocolate sun cups are fabulous!

Made Good
madegoodfoods.com/us

These are some yummy granola bars free from many allergens.

No Whey! Foods
www.nowheychocolate.com

This company makes allergy-friendly foods. We order treats from this site for Halloween and Easter!

SunButter
sunbutter.com

SunButter is a sunflower butter replacement for those with peanut allergies who cannot enjoy peanut butter. I love to carry along the individual pack for a quick snack or spread this on toast with honey for breakfast.

Tofutti
www.tofutti.com

Tofutti products are all dairy-free. I like their sour cream, cream cheese, and of course, their ice cream! As their name suggests, their products are mostly made with tofu, so if you have a soy allergy, consider looking elsewhere.

MY FAVORITE RECIPES

In addition to the processed foods in the Resources section above, I wanted to share my favorite recipes to make at home. *Bon appetit!*

SNACK FOODS

Quesadillas

I personally love quesadillas for a snack. This is a good snack for kids with allergies because quesadillas can be customized to fit taste preferences and allergy restrictions.

Ingredients (serves 1):

- 1 flour tortilla
- About ½ cup shredded cheese (I prefer Daiya non-dairy cheese)
- Cooked chicken, beef, tofu, black beans, or any other fillings you like

Directions:

1. Put the tortilla on a plate.

2. Spread fillings over half the tortilla.

3. Fold the other half over.

4. Microwave for 30 seconds to 1 minute, or cook in a skillet until the tortilla is brown and the cheese is melted.

5. Cut into triangles and enjoy! It's also tasty to dip into your favorite salsa.

If you're ready for a more challenging recipe, try this next one.

Carne Empanadas

I personally love empanadas. In the summer before seventh grade, I took my first trip to Argentina. There I had a ton of empanadas. They were delicious and allergen-free! Like the quesadilla recipe, you can also experiment with other ingredients in the empanadas.

Empanadas take a good amount of time to make, but they're worth it. First, I tried making my own dough, but now I use the Goya discs. I like to double this recipe and freeze some in a Ziploc bag after they're baked. They are great reheated in a toaster oven or microwave.

Ingredients (makes about 12 empanadas):

- 2 hard-boiled eggs chopped up (optional if you are allergic to eggs)
- Frozen Goya *discos para empanadas*
- 1 lb. ground beef
- Salt and pepper
- Olive oil
- 2 garlic cloves
- 1 tablespoon paprika
- ¼ cup pitted green olives
- 1 cup diced onion
- 1 tablespoon tomato paste
- Large pinch cayenne pepper
- Vegetable shortening, butter, or non-dairy margarine

Directions:

1. Take the Goya discs from the freezer.

2. Make the filling: Put the beef, onions, garlic, and a little olive oil (1–2 tablespoons) in the same skillet. Add pepper and salt. Sauté until meat is thoroughly cooked.

3. Stir in tomato paste, cayenne pepper, and about a cup of water.

4. Remove from stove. Stir in the olives and eggs.

5. Heat oven to 375 degrees.

6. Line a large baking sheet with parchment paper.

7. On a cutting board dusted with flour, take a disc and put about 1 ½ tablespoons of filling on half the disc, leaving a little room around the edge.

8. Fold the disc over. Use a fork to smash the two sides together. It should look like a mini calzone.

9. Place the empanada on the baking sheet (about 1 inch apart) and repeat the process until you've used all your filling.

10. You can brush the tops of the empanadas with some lard or butter. This makes them look better when they're finished, but is optional.

11. Bake for about 15 minutes or until the pastry looks crispy and golden. You should serve them warm.

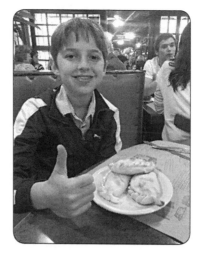

THE REAL DEAL IN BUENOS AIRES!

Hint: Serve either of these "snack" recipes with a salad and you've got a meal!

My go-to snack:

One of my other favorite snacks is a banana or an apple and SunButter. Now that you can buy individual containers of SunButter, this is a snack I can take with me to eat between school and soccer practice.

BREAKFAST

My mom won a blue ribbon at her local fair when she was my age with this recipe!

Nana's Banana Bread

Ingredients (makes 1 loaf):

- 3 ripe/overripe bananas (4 if they're small)
- ¾ cup sugar
- 1 egg
- 1 teaspoon baking soda
- 1 ½ cups flour
- ¼ cup melted butter or margarine (I use Earth Balance non-dairy)
- 1 teaspoon salt

Directions:

1. Heat oven to 325 degrees.
2. Mash bananas with a fork.
3. Stir in other ingredients.
4. Pour into a loaf pan. Bake for 50–60 minutes or until a knife inserted into the dough comes out clean.

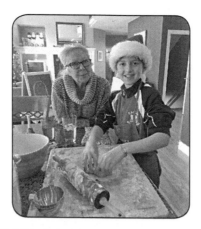

THIS IS MY GRANDMOTHER FROM FRANCE.
WE BAKE A LOT OF COOKIES AT CHRISTMAS!

Ready-to-Go Oatmeal

I help my mom make this at least once a week. She's not a morning person, so she loves to get up and know that breakfast is ready to grab!

Ingredients (makes 1 serving):

- ½ cup oats
- 1 tablespoon honey
- 1 tablespoon chia seeds
- ⅔ cup milk of your choice

Directions:

1. The night before, combine all ingredients in a large cereal bowl. Stir well.

2. Cover with plastic wrap and refrigerate.

3. In the morning, serve with fresh berries on top.

DINNER

Crepes

This is one of my family's favorite meals! Crepes work for just about anyone because each person can put in what they like. We make savory ones for dinner and sweet crepes for dessert!

Note: The batter needs to be made in advance. You can make it as little as an hour ahead of time or even the night before. The number of crepes you can make for this recipe depends on how big you make each one.

Ingredients (servings vary):
- 2 cups milk (we use soy)
- 2 eggs

- ½ teaspoon salt
- 1 ½ cups flour
- 6 tablespoons melted non-dairy margarine (or regular butter)
- Various fillings

Directions:

1. Blend the milk, eggs, and salt in a blender for 10 seconds.

2. Add the flour and blend another 30 seconds.

3. Add the melted margarine and blend for 10 more seconds.

4. Next, put the blender directly in the refrigerator to chill for at least an hour.

5. While you wait, prepare the fillings. These are the fillings we usually have, which allows everyone to mix and match what they like:

Savory Crepe Fillings:

- Cut-up deli ham
- Shredded cheese (Swiss is common in France, but I use Daiya's mozzarella)
- Cooked, sliced mushrooms

- Cooked spinach (squeeze out the liquid)
- Smoked salmon
- Crème fraiche (I use Tofutti sour cream)

Dessert Crepe Toppings:
- Sugar and butter
- Fruit of your choice (we like strawberries and bananas)
- Chocolate sauce
- Caramel sauce
- Chocolate/nut spreads (Nutella is very popular in France, but we obviously don't serve that at my house!)

6. To make the crepes, heat a small, non-stick skillet and spray with cooking spray.

7. Check the batter. Crepes are supposed to be *very* thin. If your batter is too thick, add some milk.

8. Pour the batter into the pan and add fillings on one half. Fold crepe over and cook until both sides are browned.

9. For dessert, cook crepes with no filling and serve with toppings.

If you can cook more than one crepe at a time, that is ideal. We have two crepe pans. We recently got serious and bought two crepe pans that each cook four at a time right at the table! We saw this at my cousin's in France this summer.

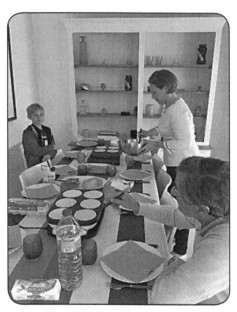

MY COUSIN MAKING SPECIAL
NON-DAIRY CREPES ON A SEPARATE
PAN FOR ME IN FRANCE.

Pasta Salad

This is another great meal for those of us with food allergies because you can put your favorite, safe foods in it. Below is one of my favorite combinations, but feel free to get creative, even with the type of pasta used.

Ingredients (makes 6 main course portions):
- 1 box fusilli pasta
- 1 diced red pepper
- 4 scallions, chopped
- 1 cup diced carrots
- 1 cup sliced mushrooms
- 1 ½ cups cherry tomatoes cut in half
- ¼ cup capers
- 1 can tuna, drained
- 1 teaspoon dried oregano
- Chopped fresh basil (as much as you like)
- 1 lemon
- Olive oil
- Salt and pepper

Directions:
1. Cook pasta according to instructions on the package and let cool.

2. Add all the ingredients through the basil.

3. Now, whisk the juice from one lemon with about ¼ cup of olive oil and salt and pepper to taste.

4. Toss this with the pasta and vegetables.

5. Serve immediately or chill until serving.

Alternatively, you can use your favorite Italian bottled dressing instead of the lemon and oil.

Chopped Salad

This is a yummy side dish or light dinner. You can adjust the veggies according to what you like.

Ingredients:

- 1 cup thawed frozen corn
- 1 can black beans (drained)
- 1 diced red pepper
- 2 celery stalks, diced
- 3 green onions, sliced
- 1 avocado
- For the dressing:
- About 2 tablespoons fresh lemon juice

- 1 tablespoon whole grain mustard
- 2–3 tablespoons olive oil

Directions:

1. Put all the salad ingredients in a bowl.

2. In a small bowl, whisk the dressing ingredients together.

3. Pour dressing over the salad and toss gently.

DESSERT

Mama's Chocolate Cake

This is a cake we make at our house a lot because it's easy and delicious!!

Ingredients:
- 1 ¾ cup flour
- 2 cups sugar
- ¾ cup cocoa
- 1 ½ teaspoons baking soda
- 1 ½ teaspoons baking powder
- 1 teaspoon salt
- 2 eggs

- 1 cup milk of your choice
- ½ cup vegetable oil
- 2 teaspoons vanilla
- 1 cup hot water (nearly boiling)

Directions:

1. Grease and flour a Bundt cake pan. Preheat oven to 325 degrees.

2. In a large bowl, whisk together flour, sugar, cocoa, baking soda, baking powder, and salt.

3. Add in eggs, milk, oil, and vanilla. Beat the mixture.

4. Stir in hot water.

5. Pour batter into Bundt pan.

6. Bake about 50 minutes, then cool before removing from pan.

THE FINAL WORD

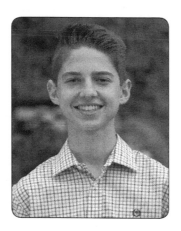

Well, there you have it! My story about my food allergies. I hope you can take it and learn from what I've done; learn from the mistakes I've made, but also take my best tips and use them in your everyday life.

I get it, food allergies are a pain in the butt, but we have to deal with them. Every time we eat, we risk our lives, but that's how it is. Mistakes WILL happen. We have to be prepared for them. In the meantime, live with caution but *live*. Travel, play sports, go to parties with your friends. Hopefully, you can even find your own way to enjoy food.

It's important we keep talking about allergies to raise awareness and support one another.

If you ever want to ask me questions or talk to me, follow me on my social media. I will be happy to get back to you. Together we can work towards making the world safer for people with food allergies.

Ciao y suerte!

—OLIVIER
Instagram: @thereal_olivier
Twitter: @allergicteen1
WhenEveryBiteMatters.com

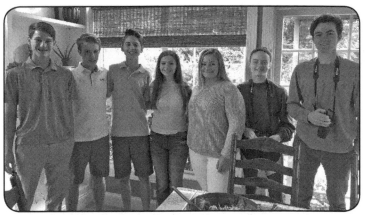

FRIENDS COMING TO THE RESCUE FOR A COVER PHOTO!

ACKNOWLEDGEMENTS

There have been many people who have helped me along the way coping with my allergies and writing this book.

I'm grateful to my family in Syracuse: Mom, Dad, Mathias & Sebastian; in France: Nana D, Dada, David, Adrien, Maxime, Mathieu & Charlie; in Missouri: Nana & Papa and Texas: Aunt Mimi, Joe, Julianna & Michael.

I'm thankful for the support of Christian Brothers Academy especially Mr. Keough, Lori Walker, Kaylie Kresse, Ms. Kenific and Ms. Stedman. From safe food at lunch to helping me start FAAB, you have allowed me to advocate for students.

Thank you, Dr. Sotomayor for being my doc and encouraging me to write this book!

This book would not look nearly as good without the help of my editor, Jessica Hatch from Hatch Editorial Services and the designer Shannon Bodie of BookWise Design. You were patient dealing with a first-time, teenage author!!

Autumn and Nathan, it was fun to create our first book cover photo together.

Finally, a big shout out to all my friends, in particular Thomas, Gabby, Liv & Jonah who are always there to help me out.

Made in the USA
Middletown, DE
27 May 2019